New Joints
and
Other Mixed Blessings

How to use prehab and rehab
to get the most
from orthopedic procedures

Jacqueline Wolfe, BA, LMT

New Joints and Other Mixed Blessings:
How to use prehab and rehab to get
the most from orthopedic procedures

Copyright 2012 by Jacqueline Wolfe

Published by
Mixed Blessings
PO Box 611
Waldport, OR 97394

Photos by Ray Winward and Jacqueline Wolfe

Printed by LAZERQUICK, Newport, Oregon, USA

ISBN Number: 978-1-480002-11-1

Library of Congress Control Number: 2012945918

1. Author: Wolfe,Jacqueline
2. Book-Health
3. Book-Self-Health Techniques
4. Joint replacement - Exercise therapy - Popular works.
5. Orthopedic surgery - Preparation - Popular works.

FIRST EDITION - 2012

Acknowledgements

I want to give a very belated thank you to Tom Fell who, in 1977, was my first and best weight lifting coach and trainer in New York City. He steered me to solid, timeless information that taught me to pay attention to, and listen to my body, while trusting myself to discern what made sense to me. I also want to thank my first martial arts instructors, Tom Bisio and Mia Wolff. In different ways they both modeled for me how education, intuition and experience work together to inform the evolution of personal health.

Thank you to all my personal training and massage clients, through whom I learned about other bodies and what affects them. A special appreciation to Patty Glas, Mary Locker, Linda Morrow, Jules Straus, Joan Wesley and Ray Winward for participating in my short class for testing the exercises in this book. These gracious and patient friends were also instrumental in helping me articulate some of the issues and difficulties that arise when working with different bodies. My appreciation to Diane Strom, of Diane's Fitness in Waldport, Oregon, for generously allowing me to use her fine space and equipment to conduct the class.

My reviewers and editors were brave, honest and generous with their time and varied expertise. John Baker; Claire Barton, PT; Patty Egan, LMT; I.F. Kelly, MA,DC; Ron Lovell, Fran Morse, Daisy Stoutsenberger, RN,P.A.c, ret., Fellow ASBP; Ruth Werner, LMT; Don Whitaker and Ray Winward - you helped to bring consistency and cohesion to this book. Thank you.

Thanks to friends, family and community, all of whom gave me encouragement and challenge as appropriate.

Finally, my very loving and supportive husband, Ray Winward, was a great part of my inspiration and participated in the process at every step. He challenged, nudged, critiqued and volunteered hands on, all the while maintaining he just wants to carry my bags. Thank you, darling.

CONTENTS

Introduction:
Why Do We Need This Book? ...………………………………… i

1. How To Use This Book ...……………………………………… 1

2. Exercises Listed, Illustrated and Explained ...…………… 3

3. Personalize Your Exercises ...………………...……………19

4. Know and Set Your Goals ...……………………………… 31

    Goal-Setting Questionnaire ...……………………………33

5. What Do We Know About Pain? ...…………………………… 37

6. Let's Understand Balance and Proprioception ...………… 45

7. Let's Talk About Self-Image ...……………………………… 49

8. Build Your Support System ...……………………………… 51

9. Tools To Help You ...………………………………………… 55

GLOSSARY ...…………………………………………………61

INDEX ...……………………………………………………64

INTRODUCTION

Why do we need this book?

I began this book as a guide for individuals preparing for, or recovering from, orthopedic surgeries. I have since realized that the ideas and exercises here can be helpful to most anyone who is not happy with their own level of physical function. The tone of the book is still aimed towards *prehab* and *rehab*, however I hope that it can serve as a meaningful guide for many others.

Working as a massage therapist over the past 16 years, I have had several clients who have had joint replacements and surgeries and have not experienced the benefits they expected from the surgery. The single biggest complaint is feeling off balance physically. Others still have pain in the area surrounding the joint long after physical therapy is over. Many retain the limps and other awkward movement patterns they developed before they had surgery. I also look back on my experiences as a personal trainer (beginning in 1978) and recognize many commonalities in people's attitudes towards their bodies and the ways in which their bodies function.

We suffer from a lack of appropriate relationship with our bodies. Many cultural attitudes and habits lead to this situation, from having lower societal priorities on physical work, to our expecting medical and insurance specialists to make the biggest and most important decisions about how we treat our bodies. But I find many astute writers bringing great insights to the issues behind this disconnect from our bodies.

In introducing a paper he is writing on his website, Anatomytrains.com, Thomas Meyers talks about bringing a measure of physical intelligence (Kinesthetic Quotient-KQ) into general conversation with the more commonly accepted Intellectual (IQ) and Emotional (EQ)s. He uses the term *"kinesthetic dystonia"* for this general ignorance about movement and the pain, reduced function, alienation, and misunderstanding that often follow.

He continues, *"For most of us educated in the Western world between 1700 and the present, however, education beyond the age of six consists of holding the kinesthetic sense as still as possible at wooden desks while the eyes and ears are over-stimulated with data. This enforced rigidity is punctuated by short periods of kinesthetic mayhem called "recess". If one is "lucky", one is released from the kinesthetic imprisonment in the afternoon for a period called "gym class", where heavy emphasis is laid on repetitive tasks and competitive sports, and rarely on art or self-discovery....*

This epidemic [of kinesthetic dystonia] comes about because we persist in "industrial" methods of educating our children about how to live in a body, and we need to develop approaches more in keeping with the requirements of the new era [of being physical persons in a largely non physically demanding world]. *A person is taught how to live in his or her body from conception onward, and we are therefore required to rework our entire idea of somatic or physical education (PE) from the ground up."*

Eli Thompson, a certified teacher of Anatomy Trains wrote,
"Is phys ed just about sports or should there be more to it? Perhaps it should be about educating our children about how to use their physical bodies more effectively in everything they do.
Our educational system emphasizes the importance of preparing children mentally and intellectually for adulthood, but not physically. Handicapped by a lack of sensory education, they misuse their bodies in most of their actions. And like fish swimming in water, they have little sense of the effort and strain being created because they are so accustomed to it."

So if you feel out of touch with your physical self and its relationship to your environment, you are not alone. Most adults in our North American culture have grown up through a system that is not kinesthetically user friendly.

All human systems, however, are pretty resilient. Our brains and minds have a wonderful characteristic called plasticity. This means that we can learn and adapt - at any age. So whether you are interested in adapting a little or a lot, I hope you will find this book to be a helpful start.

One of the goals of this book is to suggest a variety of options for pain-free, but effective, exercises that will allow most individuals to find a safe way to gain improved function and understanding in their own bodies. This would have the benefit of making the long-term results of any orthopedic surgery more successful.

I fully expect that you will find yourself personalizing at least some part of this information as if you knew it instinctively or had already learned it at some level. We have learned to leave too much to the "experts" at the risk of ignoring what we learn about our own workings throughout our own lives.

Our economy has been slowing in recent years and may continue to do so for some time to come. We will be well served by getting and keeping as fit as we can on our own, so that we may rely less on a medical and insurance system that may not be able to keep up with our needs, especially if we continue to have long lives. The tools and insights offered here should serve as an excellent framework for keeping tabs on, and maintaining, your best health. I am not the ultimate expert, but you can be the ultimate expert of your own body. I hope I will offer some helpful discussions for you to accomplish exactly that.

CHAPTER 1

HOW TO USE THIS BOOK

If you already have a basic knowledge of exercise and have done some before, you might want to take a look at the exercises included in Chapter 2. If you have any problems with any of the exercises, please take a look at the other parts of the book where I address several of the major issues that prevent our getting the benefit we desire from moving. Not the least of these is that many of us were taught poorly or even wrongly about how to work with our own bodies. There are many, many misconceptions that still pervade our understanding of how bodies work best.

I have tried to title sections so that you can find what you want when you want it. Feel free to read out of order. Also, to paraphrase martial artist Bruce Lee, *"Take what is useful and shelve the rest."*

If you are someone who is uncomfortable after looking at these exercises, please read forward a bit more into the book. The same principles apply as for those with more experience but there are more tools available than you might know. You may want to take a look at some of the resources noted under the *Tools* chapter. Sometimes a slight variation in form or explanation can be enlightening. Some will need more self-education to begin to access these principles. I have been through this process, as has my husband. Indeed we are both still going through *joint issues* and trying to gain awareness and understanding of what we can do at our own levels. We work to be able to do what we want to do with our bodies while avoiding pain. Discovery of our bodies is an ongoing process that doesn't ever end (nor should it) until we die.

Even if you have no problem understanding and performing the exercises I recommend reading through the chapter on *Personalizing the Exercises*. I still discover attitudes and beliefs that keep me from getting the most from my work and, after some initial dismay, find the discoveries exciting.

Clients and friends (including myself and my husband) who have had less extreme orthopedic surgeries have also had varying degrees of success. Over the years I have tried to notice what conditions exist that allow such varied responses to often very similar procedures. The two most common disconnects occur in *goal setting and expectations* and in *preparation*. This whole book addresses various aspects of preparation, but knowing and setting goals is at the same time easier, and more difficult than we might expect. When you do the self-questionnaire in Chapter 4 you will understand what I mean.

CHAPTER 2

BASIC EXERCISES

TOE RAISES and CALF STRETCHES

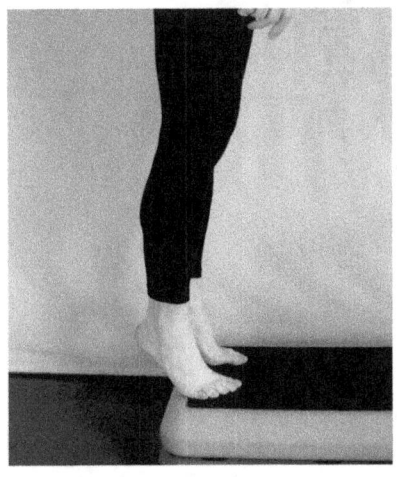 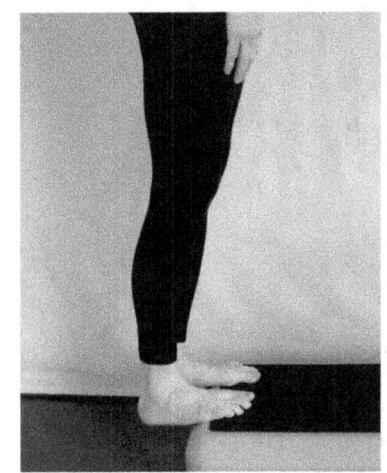

Stand on a step. (This can be the bottom step on stairs in your home, the binding side of a heavy book or something else that is firm and stable and won't tip.) Try to just use your fingertips on a wall or railing for balance. Go up onto the toes of both feet, pause for a couple of seconds then go slowly down so that your heels hang below the step. Feel what happens in every part of your feet and legs; even in your stomach and back. If this feels too easy, try doing it one leg at a time.

This exercise is one of the most basic for strength and balance, not only of the lower leg, but for the whole body. Keeping the ankles flexible and strong allows us to adapt to standing and walking on different surfaces. It is the first step in absorbing shock to save our other joints from excessive pounding.

STANDING PELVIC TILTS

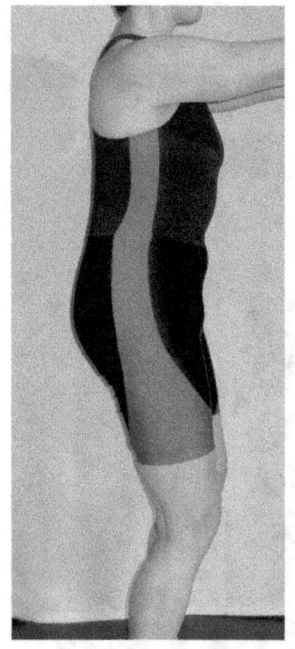 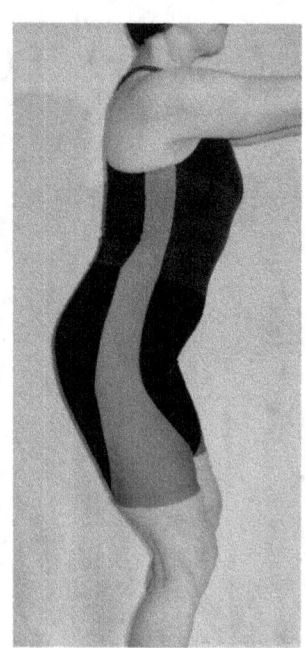

Stand with your feet flat and wide enough to feel stable, and your and knees slightly bent. Tuck your tail bone under so that your groin area moves forward. Then rock your tail bone back so your lower back arches like you're sticking your butt out. Though your knees are flexed a bit, keep the movement in your hips. Once you get the feel of the movement try to make it smoother, rather than jerking from front to back.

When we learn this movement, it is usually from a lying down position. I think it is important to be aware of how the movement feels when we are supporting ourselves against gravity. You can also do this exercise sitting or lying down to increase and maintain mobility in the pelvis.

This is an excellent place to introduce what we will be calling your "core." The muscles in the area around our lower stomach, low back, hips and into our groin area (pelvic floor) are often referred to as our "core" muscles.

NECK STRETCH ROTATION   **NECK SIDEBENDING**

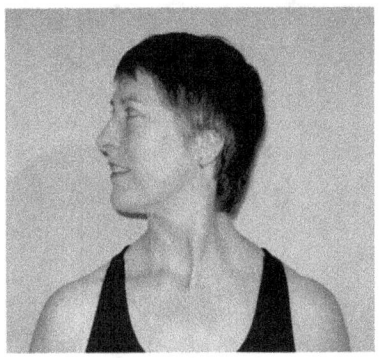
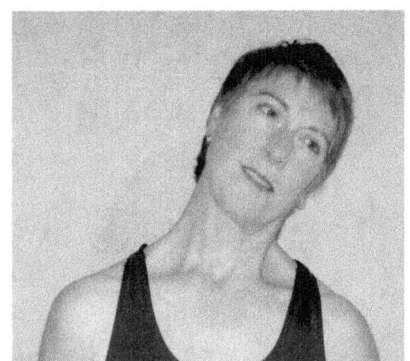

NECK ROTATION

Sitting comfortably, pull your shoulder blades slightly back and rotate your head to one side as far as comfortable without sticking your chin out. Stop and note how this feels to you. Use your neck muscles on the side to which you're turning to hold the position. Take a slow breath, look behind you with your eyes and pause, then, only with the eyes, look forward. (Don't go so far that it hurts your eyes.) Take another slow breath then look backwards again and see if you can turn your head a bit more.

Slowly turn your head to the front, take a breath, then repeat the stretch to the other side. It is important to take these movements slowly.

NECK SIDEBENDING

Face your head to the front, take a breath, then bend your head toward one shoulder. Make sure both of your shoulders are down and slightly back. (It might be helpful to do this in front of a mirror.) Take a couple of slow breaths in this position, moving a bit this way or that, as feels good. Again, use your neck muscles on the side you're bending *toward* to help. Bring your head back to the center and breathe slowly. Repeat to the right...slow...

The neck work stretches muscles that can often restrict your breathing when they are tight. Strengthening these muscles and keeping them flexible can help make your breathing be more efficient and help save strain on the whole back. We tend to tighten these muscles with most exertion and they are often responsible for a myriad of headaches. If we become aware of them through moving and stretching them, we have a much greater chance of being able to relax them when needed.

TORSO ROTATIONS

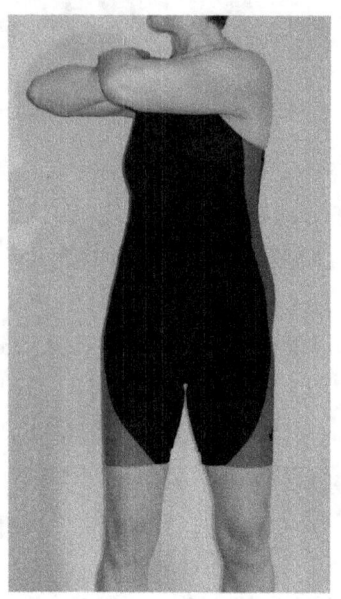 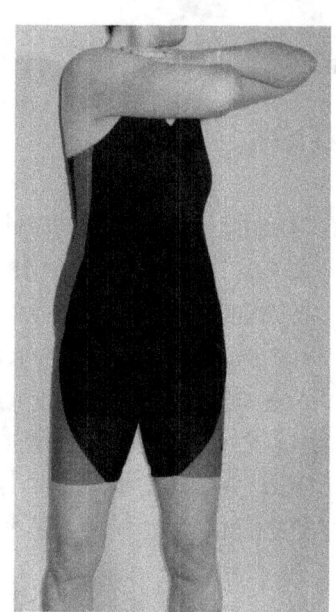

Stand with your feet flat and in a wide stance, or sit with your arms folded across your shoulders. Rotate your torso to one side, keeping your hips facing front. Hold for a few seconds then repeat to the other side. Try this in front of a mirror so you can see your hip position. Don't worry about how far you can turn. It almost always feels farther than it looks.

This is for middle (thoracic) and upper torso mobility – NOT the lower back (lumbar) area. Be sure to keep your hips facing forward with your pelvis tucked while doing this, and allow the arms to help you.

BENT KNEE RAISE

STRAIGHT LEG KNEE RAISE

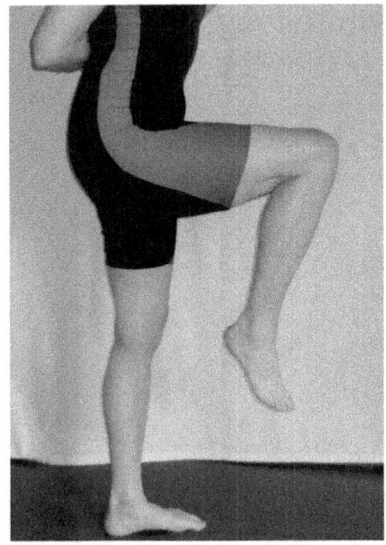

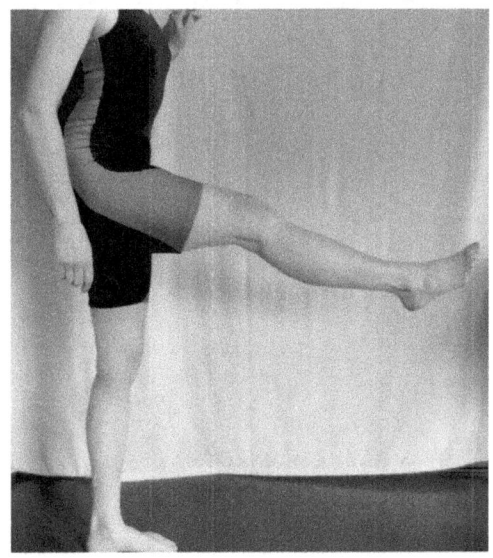

BENT

March in place or lift one bent leg at a time. If you can't get your knee very high, try tucking your pelvis under and lengthening your back. If bending your knee is a problem, just bend it as much as you can. Your movement may be more like a straight front raise. Take your time with this, be aware of how your standing leg feels and stay as upright as you can. Feel free to hold onto something for balance if you need to.

This works on improving hip mobility, and, believe it or not, also works your stomach muscles.

STRAIGHT

Standing, lift one straight leg to the front with a tightened knee. Repeat with the other leg. Feel free to use a wall or railing to help balance, but try to use just fingertips. Engage your core muscles for balance and support by trying not to lean back. Don't worry about how high you lift your leg.

This exercise is great if you have knee pain that prevents you from bending and straightening at the knee. It strengthens the quadriceps muscles that move the knee from the front of the thigh, as well as the muscles that flex the hips, while lengthening the hamstrings and other muscles at the back of the leg.

BACKWARD LEG RAISE WITH BENT KNEE

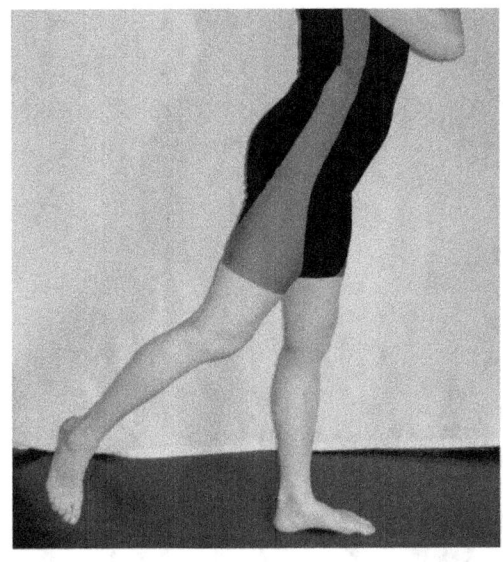 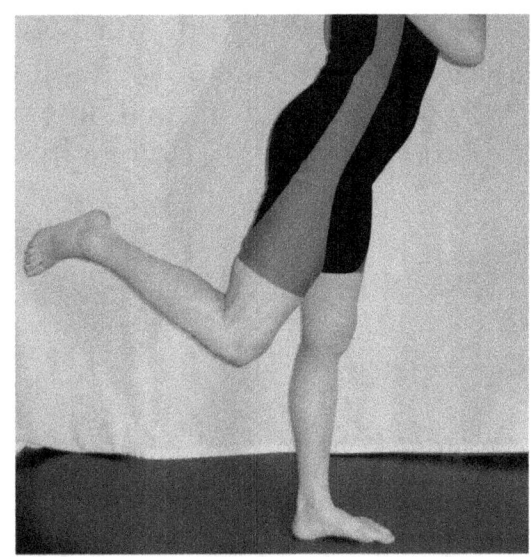

STRAIGHT

While standing, face a wall or railing. Remain as upright as possible and raise one leg behind you. Keep your leg as straight as possible, though it may feel better for you if you bend your leg. Sometimes it helps to push away with the heel.

This exercise strengthens the buttocks and low back, but make sure you are conscious of not straining your low back. You might not be able to take your leg very high. Most people can't. If you feel tension in your low back, you might be arching there. If so, drop your chin, your chest and your leg just enough to feel your buttocks tighten without straining your low back. Be conscious of using your core to support you. You may lean a bit forward by bending your arms into the wall, just not so far that you don't feel your backside working. This also helps stretch the hip flexors which are in the front of the hip. Many people have very tight hip flexors from excessive sitting and lack of movement. This usually causes bent or stooped posture and an inability to lift the legs much, resulting in a shuffling gait.

BENT

Same as the back leg lift, but now try to bend your leg first, then lift from the butt. If your hamstring muscles in the back of the thigh start to cramp take the leg lower. This has the same benefits as the straight lift, but gives a better stretch to the quadriceps in the front of the thigh. It also works the hamstrings to strengthen those muscles that bend the knee.

STANDING HIP HIKE

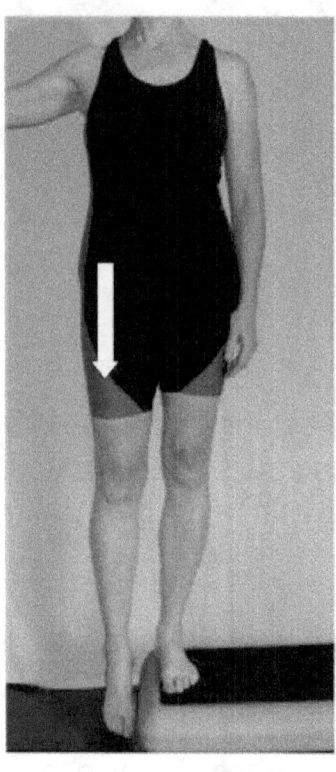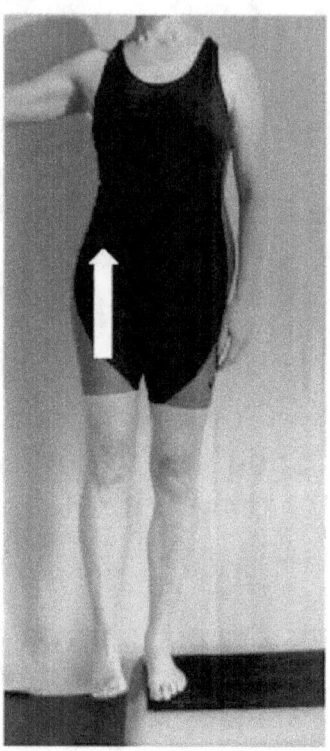

Stand on a step and let your outside leg hang off the step. Keeping your hanging leg straight, hike that outside hip up, then let it down again, trying not to rock your body much from side to side. This is a tiny movement. Try to make it smooth, not jerky.

I recommend this especially for those who have pain when using the hip joint. The muscles that perform most of this hip "hike" are the gluteus medius in the pelvis and the quadratus lumborum in the low back. Strengthening and using these muscles can help protect from some of the pounding that occurs when walking.

HIP WHEELS

You might want to try a more advanced form of this movement by taking your hip to the front and back, as well as up and down, (as if your hip and leg were a vehicle wheel). This more closely resembles what the hip does when walking fluidly. Remember it is always fine to use a wall or railing for balance.

This adds even more mobilization to the pelvis, which integrates the whole hip structure. It sounds odd, but this movement can help you to limp more effectively, or to recognize the mechanisms of limping when you are trying to get rid of a limp.

SETTING SHOULDERS

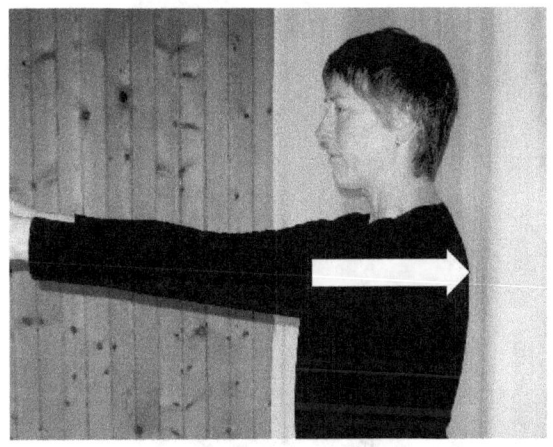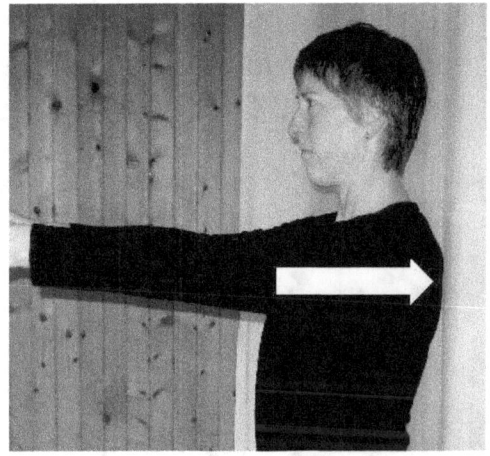

Stand with your back and head (if possible) against a wall. Raise your arms straight in front of you at about 90 degrees. Without moving anything else stretch your arms as far as they will go. Now, moving your shoulder blades only, pull your arms/shoulders back to the wall. The shoulders go back, but the shoulder blades don't pull together. Remember this feeling. This is another tiny movement.

Whenever you lift with your arms or put weight into your shoulders, you should first set the shoulder blades. This is the best way to support the less stable shoulder joint. It's importance can't be stressed enough. This is how you should feel when you stand up straight, rather than jutting your chest out.

SEATED LEGS LIFT

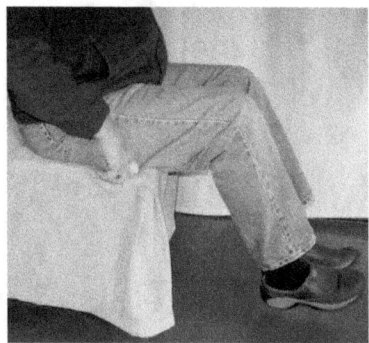

Sit on a firm chair with your legs bent 90 degrees and lift both feet an inch or so off the floor. Don't arch your low back, but rather tighten your stomach by pulling it into your back. This strengthens the stomach (and the front of the legs).

You can do this by lifting one foot at a time to get the correct feel. Once you feel your stomach engaging, move to lifting both feet. remember to just lift an inch or so.

SPIDER

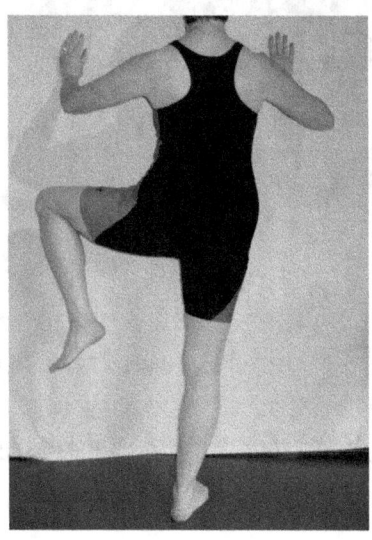 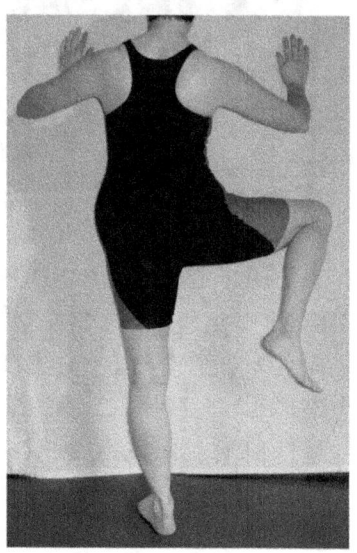

Facing a wall, set your shoulders and lean into the wall. Bring one bent leg up the same side of your body, as if trying to reach your elbow like a spider. As in several other exercises, this movement may actually be rather small. Repeat with the other leg.
This works lateral abdominal muscles and hips.

HUDDLE STRETCH

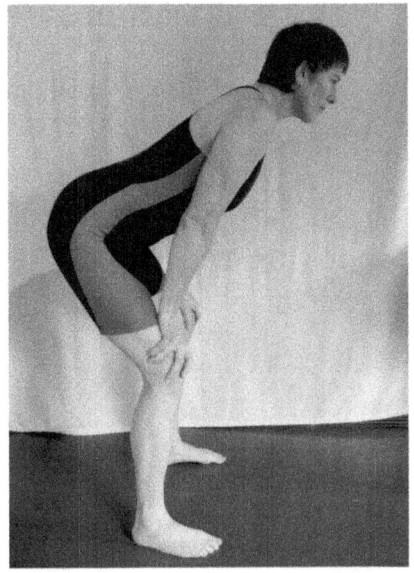 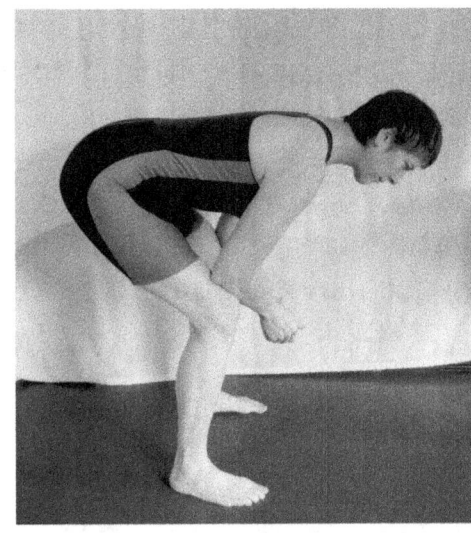

With a wide stance, bend your knees slightly and place your hands or elbows on your knees. Feel the controlled, supported stretch in your back. This is a good preparation for getting down to the floor.

WALK IN PLACE

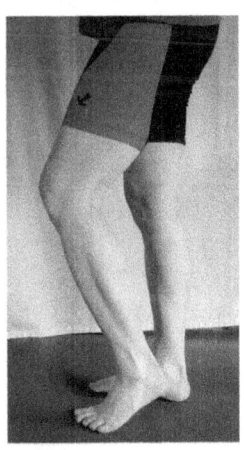 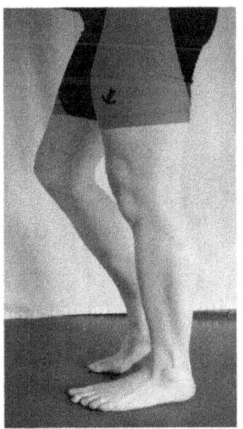

Keep both feet *on the floor* and go up on each toe alternately as the other foot stays flat. Exaggerate hip movement to each side with a little bounce. Use your arms by moving them with the hips, however don't let them cross in front of your body.

You can make this a more advanced movement by rotating the hips in a figure eight, but still keep the arms from crossing in front of the body. This may be difficult to imagine, but once you try it, it should make more sense.

This also works at mobilizing your hips. (If you can't get the coordination down at first just send your hips side-to side by bending each knee.) Don't forget to move your arms - that helps with balance.

WALL PLANK

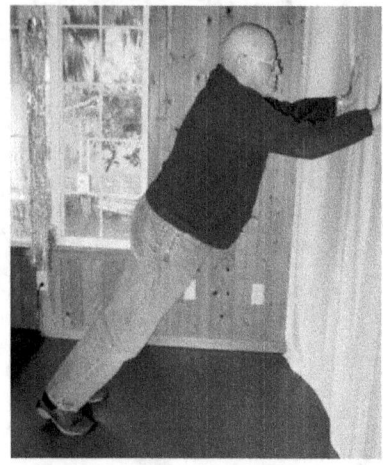

Lean into a wall as if you were preparing to do a push-up. With head up and chin in, use your stomach muscles to keep your middle from sagging. This helps strengthen the core muscles. A more advanced exercise would be to lean into a lower bench or chair.

SIT ON BALANCE BALL (See tools chapter on how and where to purchase.)

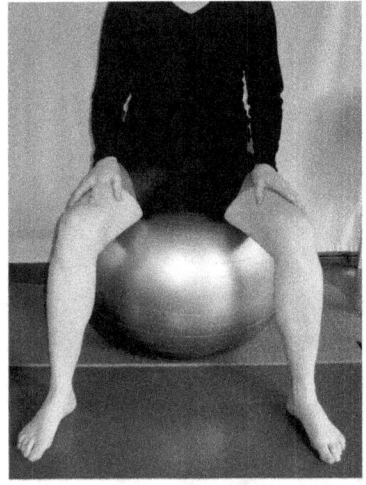 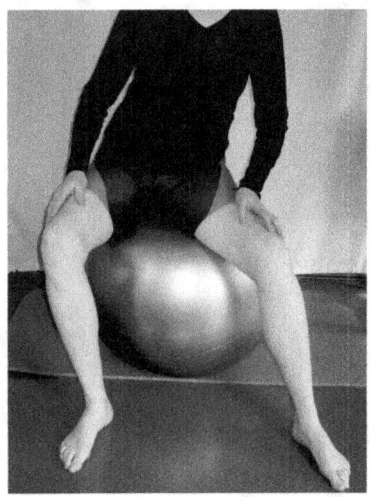 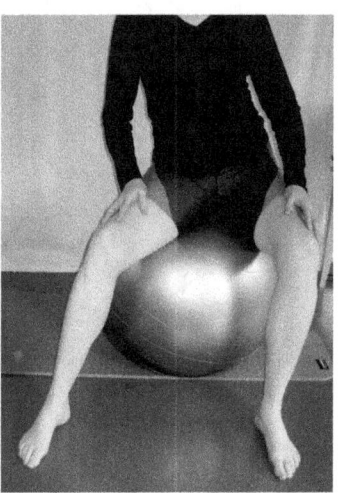

Sit on a properly inflated balance ball with your feet and legs spread wide. Even though this may feel unfamiliar and uncomfortable for many women this wide stance allows you a very stable base - like a triangle.

Move your hips side to side. Then try moving forward and back by bending and straightening your legs. Remember these are small movements that can feel huge. Feel the difference with your feet closer together and farther apart. When you feel balanced try a little bounce, then a bit more. Practice rising and sitting without using your hands, then without bouncing. Feel free to do this in front of a rail or table where you can hold on if needed.

This is an excellent exercise from which to start feeling how you move from your center of gravity. The muscles in the area around your lower stomach, low back, hips and into your groin area (pelvic floor) are often referred to as your "core" muscles. Being in touch with these muscles, being able to keep them strong and using them to help move can make your life easier and more comfortable in many ways.

RISE FROM CHAIR WITHOUT USING HANDS

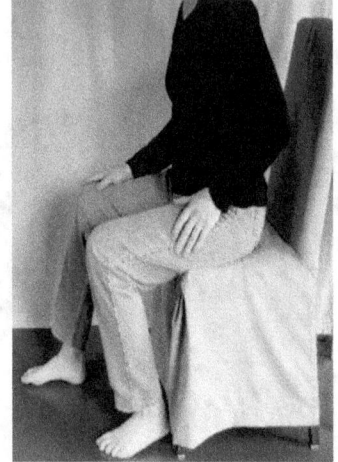 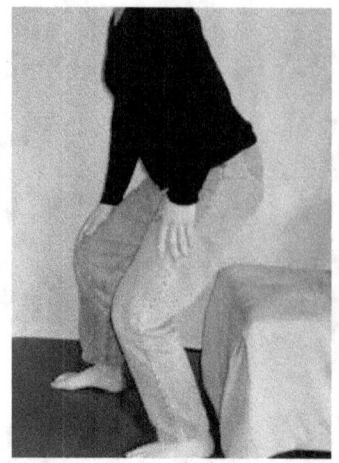

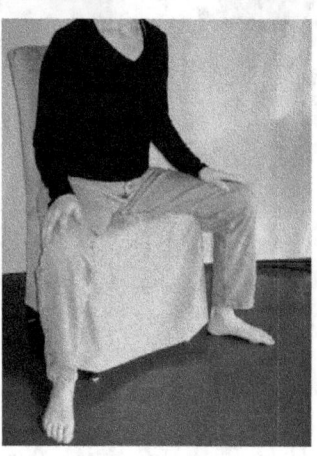 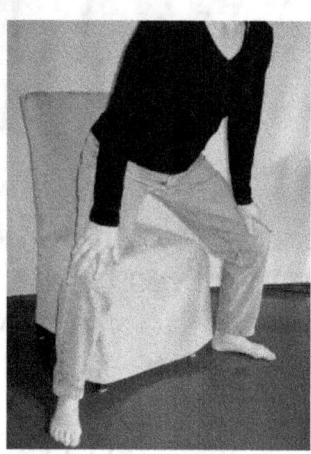

Sit in a chair that is solid and high enough to allow your thighs to be fairly parallel to the floor. Most people do better with one foot well in front of the other and fairly wide apart. Lean forward and LIFT yourself FORWARD and up without using your hands. If you have flexible hips you can just spread your legs wide and LIFT (lower photos). Take the weight out of your hands if you can, and lift from your core (like squeezing to stop your urine flow).

If you were able to do the balance ball exercise, use what you learned from that to do this. (note: It's not just from bouncing, but from preparing, setting or *pre-loading* our muscles.) This movement does wonders to strengthen core muscles and to integrate movement from your feet up through the rest of your body. Feel free to do this in front of a rail or table where you can reach forward or hold on if needed.

HIP WALKS

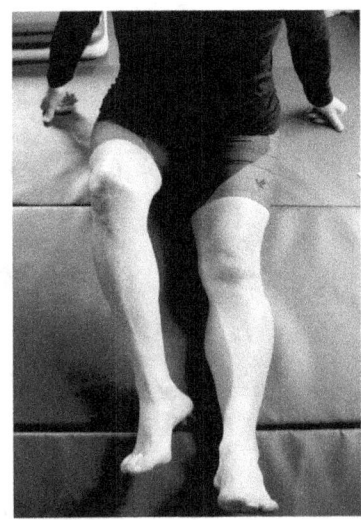 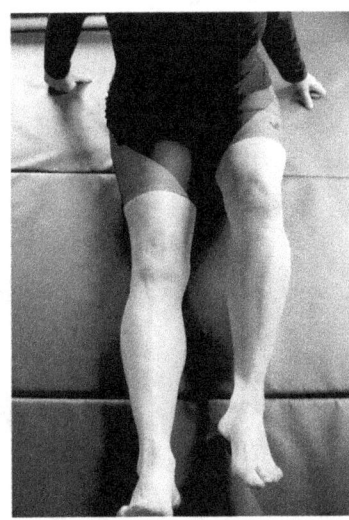

This exercise is best felt sitting on the floor but you *can* do it sitting in a chair with your feet up on another chair. Move your hips back and forth, then walk yourself forwards and backwards on your butt. You will rock a bit side to side, but try to actually lift one sitz bone and move it forward like one of those old wind-up toys. Believe it or not, the way we do this on the floor is exactly how our hips should move when we walk on our feet.

Often the hardest part of this is getting down to the floor. This exercise is all about mobilizing your hips.

AND MORE...?

Eventually you may move to more advanced exercises like lowering to, and rising from the floor, as well as doing exercises on the floor. These might also include stretches for the back of the legs and the low back, as well as for the front of the body and the hip flexors. More complex movements are more difficult to illustrate, and might be better shown on video. I will attempt to do that on my website.

Hopefully the following chapters will help you set your own goals for your future and help you accomplish them.

All of these exercises work on balance and proprioception-*knowing where your body parts are in space and in relation to the rest of your body*. This helps with fluidity of movement and thus security in motion.

It is important to be able to accommodate movements so you can do them as comfortably as possible.

It is ALWAYS acceptable to have something stable nearby to grab in case you lose your balance.

Having a friend or group to do these exercises with you can be invaluable for several reasons:

⅄   Encouragement and compliance (to make sure you both DO the exercises and help make corrections)

⅄   Give each other feedback, share your discoveries and commiserate

⅄   For a safety back-up

CHAPTER 3

Personalize Your Exercises

The exercises in the previous chapter may seem so basic they may not seem like real exercises. However they address conditions, like not being able to rise from a chair without using your hands, or "falling" into chairs instead of sitting. These conditions are not considered normal in assessing the mobility and balance of older adults. It is my hope after reading this chapter, you will have the feeling you already knew the information. I'm sure you already do, at least at some level. Many people have learned to ignore their instincts in favor of what "experts" espouse and to accept being less mobile than they desire. I hope to present enough information here to encourage you to trust yourself in how you improve your ability to move and get stronger.

Over the past few decades there have been numerous television shows and books that make promises that their way is the only real way to look or be fit. Many of these programs are about how we *look*, with little, if any, respect for how we function in our daily lives. Often this information is accepted for years as holy truth. At the same time new information that is more scientifically current takes a long time to enter the mainstream.

We do have a lot to learn from fitness science which, perhaps by definition, tends to be targeted at the young and usually those who are already fit. Some of the all-time best information about our bodies and how they work has come from sports medicine. Because sports physiology targets *optimum* performance, rather than mere physical competence, the science asks targeted questions at a very high level. There is probably more understanding of the diversity of individual physiologies and physiques arising from this field than from any other. However it still learns from and addresses the young and fit.

When I began looking for exercises or modalities that might help benefit my older clients who were not well-served by the current offerings I found virtually nothing. Even Tai Chi was too strenuous for many of them. There are some great systems out there, but for many individuals those systems need to be significantly modified to what might be considered starting at zero.

Then Let's Start at Zero...

A joint moves because muscles cross the joint and those muscles move bones closer to, or away from, each other. Many muscles cross more than one joint. For instance, most people are aware that the muscles on the front (quadriceps) and back (hamstrings) of the thigh straighten or bend the knee. Both of these muscle groups, however, have parts that also cross the hip joint. *This gives us an alternative way to strengthen these muscles and to use the joint without causing more pain to an already compromised knee.* This is very important before and after surgery.

Much research has shown that strengthening muscles, especially those in the lower body, contributes to better balance before and after surgery and better results from the surgery itself. Our goals in doing these exercises are not restricted to strengthening specific muscles, but extend to increasing our ability to move effectively, especially in ways that have become difficult for us. This entails strengthening muscles, but not necessarily in the traditional way of isolating them from other muscle movements. Remember, we want to be functional.

When you do the *front leg raise* exercises you are working the quadriceps muscles with minimal strain on the knee but, more importantly, you are integrating muscles in the hip joint to help accomplish movement of the knee. Almost every movement we do with our knees uses the hips as well, so it makes sense to consciously use the joints together.

Similarly, when you do the *bent back leg raise,* you are working the hamstrings without straining the knee. You may not be working as many parts of the muscles as if you were doing exercises that did put stress on the knee, but you are nonetheless improving your strength and balance, which allows you to keep moving the knee without causing further pain.

Almost every exercise can be modified to accommodate the fitness level and pain tolerance of individual needs. When starting out, don't worry about how many repetitions (reps) you do. One or two can be plenty. Feel free to try one or two at different times of the same day. Do them *slowly, consciously and with control,* because if you really hurt you probably won't try again.

I have also found that many movements are difficult simply because we haven't done them before. Even an accomplished athlete will often feel uncoordinated and sore after doing a different workout than one they are used to. I have observed that most people get a movement or exercise down to their comfort level after about three tries. By then, your nervous system will know what to expect and your balance will be better. If you pay attention to yourself, you will know what muscles to use and how to recruit them for each movement. After trying a new movement on three different occasions (approximately) you will likely be much more successful.

Success doesn't necessarily mean you will master the movement as originally tried. Sometimes we need to change how we do a movement. Often people with joint issues will find they experience pain or discomfort in an area not directly related to the movement itself. For instance, while doing the standing leg raises some people will experience pain in their *standing* knee or hip, rather than in the lifting one. If this happens you can do fewer repetitions for less time. Sometimes bending or straightening the standing leg helps. Sometimes leaning into a wall or railing or hanging onto a hanging rope can take some of the weight. *Thoughtfully modifying an exercise does not constitute cheating.*

When you need to change an exercise, the first modification is usually a smaller range of motion. If a movement feels uncomfortable, make it smaller. At the same time, you can pay close attention to the particulars of the motion. For instance, let's explore a squat, also called a knee bend. This is basically like sitting down without using your hands. And let's say that osteoarthritis is present and painful in both knees. Your first option might be to just slightly bend the knees to see how far you can go within your own pain tolerance and without losing your balance. You might spread your feet so your stance is wider. You can hold onto a railing or a table for this attempt. If you can go partway without pain, but fear going farther, try squatting onto an exercise ball or a higher chair. You may be able to do the "down" part but need help to get up. That's OK. If you have access to a hanging rope you could use that to hold onto and help you get up and down without putting all your weight on your legs.

You might even have to just imagine yourself doing a movement without actually doing it - let your brain do the movement until you feel ready. This is called *visualization*. It is an integral tool for many athletes that is used to improve and perfect performance. It can be a great tool for the rest of us too.

This attempt may actually end up being another exercise altogether. That's OK too. When you gain more function, you can always try again. So even though the exercises I've included in the previous chapter are simple, rather than complex, they too can be simplified or changed. Doing another exercise to target the same muscles as an exercise that isn't working for you takes some education. You need to know which muscles and joints are being targeted, but it can be done. That is why, instead of complex exercises that use several joints, the exercises I've listed work at focusing on using one joint at a time in the primary movement. So instead of doing squats or knee bends, you can do the backward leg raise to strengthen your hamstrings and gluteals (the muscles in the back of your thigh and in your butt). Getting up from a chair or ball works the same muscles as a squat, but with support, and focuses on your core, which is very important in squatting movements.

If you are working with a physical therapist or a personal trainer, knowing specifically *why* an exercise isn't right for you can help both of you work on finding another exercise that helps you accomplish what you want.

A recent study published in the journal *Physical Therapy* found that older adults who had trouble *Stooping, Crouching and Kneeling (SCK)* had significant decreases in strength in the muscles that straighten the knee and those that point and flex the ankle, as well as in muscles that extend (straighten) the back. They also point out in their conclusion that, *"Although muscle groups that were key to rising from SCK were examined, there are other muscle groups that may contribute to safe SCK performance."* This demonstrates that, rather than not doing a movement because of limitations, we may be able to recruit different muscles to support painful joints while still strengthening the muscles that are considered primary to a movement.

MOST COMMON ISSUES

⅄ We often unknowingly impose outside limitations upon ourselves. These include things like shoes that slip on or off our feet or that don't, for one reason or another, give enough stability. Women are more often prone to this because of appearance. If you shuffle when you walk because of pain and you also wear slides that don't allow you to take a stride without the shoes falling off, then you *must* find more appropriate footwear in order to accomplish your other goals. The same goes for tight-fitting or too-loose clothing or other clothes that don't allow you to move or breathe freely. As age challenges our abilities to move fluidly and freely, we often need to assess our comfort and mobility as much as our appearance.

⅄ A stiff *neck* can be a real nuisance and can affect balance and breathing as well. No recommended exercise should put stress on the neck. When you do neck exercises or stretches, be sure to keep your shoulders down and to breathe. Do neck movements slowly. If you don't have much range of motion in your neck, simply be aware of what your range is. If you have bony changes or arthritis that limits your range, be aware of that. If you only have tight neck muscles you can expect more improvement in range, but only to what your bones will allow. Be patient and enjoy what you can do and breathe, breathe, breathe at every step.

⅄ Arthritic *hands* can also impose limitations on your sense of balance because you might not have enough confidence in your grip or dexterity to grab a rail, break a fall or support yourself in other ways. Being aware that this condition exists and influences your fears about how you move is an important step. I find that using the flat of a soft fist is usually an acceptable option for most times when you must use your hands to support some of your weight. This position has the advantage of allowing you to keep your wrist in a strong position while also allowing pretty free positioning of crooked and spindled fingers.

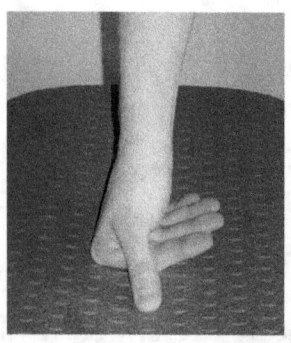 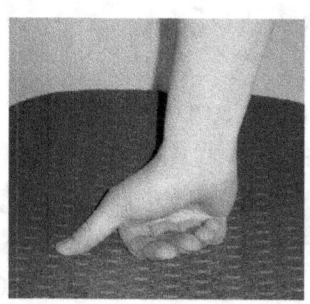

⅄ Weak or compromised *shoulders* can also affect efficient movement, especially when doing exercise. You should keep your elbows well below shoulder level and your hands closer, rather than farther from your body whenever supporting any weight, including your own. If you do this you should be able to comfortably hold onto rail or lean into a wall for support. When getting up and down, whether from a chair or the floor, you may need to have a stool, chair or table at an appropriate height to assist your movements until you develop other muscles (especially your core) to do more of the work. And learn to always set your shoulders from the shoulder blade when preparing to lift, pull, throw or otherwise stress (use) your shoulders. (see exercises.)

⅄ *Low back* pain can be debilitating and I don't pretend to know what that is like. There are many, many books dedicated to back pain and to low back pain in general. I do know, however, that the low back is the most common structural body location affected by emotion. Whether these are emotions resulting from the pain (often feelings about the pain itself) or emotions from other things that have been suppressed, consciously or unconsciously, the back suffers. All I ask is that you try small movements, bit by bit, to let the area move. Of course, it is important to check with your physician, but many doctors don't have any better understanding of your low back pain than you do. Gaining some understanding of how the pelvis moves and its important connections to the low back can also give us some amazing tools to help with the low back.

There are two things that are often misunderstood about the low back. The first is that it is not particularly flexible. The lumbar spine is made for strength and stability so, except for pre-adolescent acrobats whose bones haven't fused, most of us have limited range of movement in this area - though it is important to have *some*. The second misconception I often see is that people often arch backward and feel that they are stretching the low back by doing this. This is actually *contracting* the low back muscles. It is possible that tightening these muscles gets an infusion of fresh blood into the region, making it feel warmer and less stiff.

Leaning forward will actually stretch the low back muscles. I suggest that you not just hang your back, but rather bend the knees slightly and rest your hands or elbows on your knees (like being in a football huddle - see exercises) to control and support the stretch. Doing the stretch with no support can actually cause the muscles to tighten up because they "think" they're going to tear. More advanced exercises like hip swings and hip rocks can also be freeing for low back tension, but, as with everything else, pay attention to how *you* are feeling and work within your comfort zone. If you do so, that comfort zone will expand.

Relative to back pain, there is a technique that many find helpful in integrating what's happening to us on the surface and what's in our deep unconscious. It is called Emotional Freedom Technique (EFT) or Tapping. I will talk more about this in the chapter on *Tools*. The technique comes from a mixture of Traditional Chinese Medicine using acupressure points and modern psychotherapeutic understanding. EFT is easy to do by yourself in the privacy of your own home. I like to begin a class with it to help release any irrational self-sabotaging. EFT is also great for issues other than back pain and I will address that later.

⌀ Immobile *hips* are an American phenomenon. Free hip movement is often considered feminine and sexual. Most men don't swing their hips when they walk because that is socially considered a feminine trait. We make fun of John Wayne's gait and most literary cowboys, detectives and gangsters have a markedly "measured stride." That's too bad for them because they are often shortchanging their full range of walking motion, as women often do as well.

For women, many have been taught that swinging our hips is sexually suggestive and an invitation for "sexual" attention. High heels arch the back and restrict our ability to use our hips effectively. Social expectations have done an injustice for all of us in this respect. Walking upright is made possible by the special structure of our hips and pelvises. Because women's hips are wider than men's the angle at which the thigh bone attaches to the pelvis is more acute and causes more natural sway with movement. However, men should also have some rolling movement to their hips when ambulating. (see www.swingwalker.net. for a beautiful demo.)

Having stated the above, immobile, tight or restricted hips are as often the result of other dysfunctions as the cause of them. Rarely do they stand alone. Several of the exercises in Chapter 3 address hip movement. While for many these exercises actually feel silly, be assured that when the hips flow freely much low back pain dissipates, if not disappears altogether. Fluid hip movement can also have a positive effect on hips, knees and ankles, not to mention the joints of the upper body.

HOW HIPS WORK

As they relate to walking, the hips are made up of three bones: the *ilium* and *sacrum*, which are parts of the pelvis and form the sacroiliac joints; and the head of the *femur* (the big leg bone) which fits into the ilium, and forms the *iliofemoral* joint. This is the hip joint we address when we talk about "hip replacement." Many people develop a stride in which the iliofemoral joint is used disproportionately to the other pelvic joints. To be more fluid and effective, however, it is necessary to integrate the sacroiliac joints. It is helpful to know how these joints work together. We also need to recognize the slight rotation that occurs at the joint of the lumbar spine and the sacrum called the *sacrovertebral* joint.

A pelvis that is walking fluidly looks somewhat like a *"flexing figure 8"* lying flat on its side when looking down from above the body. Most of the muscles that actually allow us to lift our leg and put it down (forward and backward leg raise) attach to the ilium, but if we only use the motion of lifting and setting down we stay in place (walk in place). We also need to move forward and, sometimes, backward. If we do the exercises that use greater hip movement (standing hip hike, hip "wheel" rotations, hip walks, hip rocks - Pg. 12,18) we can begin to feel the integration of all of our walking hip parts. When we actually walk, the movements in the sacroiliac and sacrovertebral joints are tiny, but allow for a more fluid and dynamic stride.

Sometimes it is *pain in the standing leg* that prevents us from doing our standing hip exercises. Do them in smaller amounts, use a handhold for balance or focus on the non-standing exercises. I can't say this enough - do what you do well and with attention. The time or quantity are far less important than getting in touch with how you function.

Abdominal strength (seated legs lift, spider, wall plank) and flexibility is very important in supporting all other movements of the body. The abdominals and the pelvic floor muscles constitute what we refer to as our "core." Abdominal strength and flexibility are also imperative in preventing low back pain. Traditional sit-ups and crunches can be fun for someone who is already strong to show off, but they are not the best exercises for developing functional abdominal strength. The abdominal muscles are also some of the best muscles at recruiting other muscles to help flex the body because they are only capable of slight movement. Their primary job is stabilization. So forget doing hundreds, or even tens, of stomach exercises. Do a few, pay attention, do them well. There are more exercises for the abdominals and other muscles included in several of the resources listed at the end of this book.

Another problem with abdominals and the muscles that flex our bodies forward is that most of us spend a great deal of our time in a seated position - in flexion. That is a good reason to consciously stretch and open our fronts when we stand and when we walk. That is a good reason to do abdominal work from an upright position.

It is also our abdominal muscles that help us balance when we turn around, whether lying down, sitting or standing. When these muscles are stronger we have a much decreased risk of falling when walking or changing direction.

THE KNEE

The *knee* is the most frequently replaced joint. I suspect that most people who use this book will be dealing with knee pain at some level and many will be preparing to have total knee replacement. Many of the exercises included in the previous chapter both directly and indirectly target strengthening muscles that affect the knees. It seems ironic that knee pain might well keep you from doing some of those movements. If that happens there are a few things that I will recommend.

The first is to do fewer of the movements until you get stronger and develop better balance. The second suggestion is to change the angle of your knee slightly by bending or straightening it, even while doing an exercise. Something else you can try is to change the position of your foot by turning it in or out a bit. You will notice that the first, and maybe the most important, exercise that I listed in Chapter 3 addresses ankle strength and flexibility. That can have an immeasurable effect on your knees. Any of these factors can make a difference, but you must remember to think about and to try different suggestions before giving up. Keep reconsidering, even *after* giving up, and let the surrender be temporary.

The last suggestion I have for knees is to monitor whether you are actually feeling pain or *anticipating* pain and tightening in response. It is important is for you to be honest with yourself about this. I have done it, my husband has done it, my clients have done it. I know it happens and that is very difficult to acknowledge or admit. Just allow this awareness to be a potential part of the equation.

ANKLES AND FEET

Ankle and foot issues can affect the whole stack of bones. I have two basic suggestions here: change the position of your feet, one foot at a time, or both together. Turn them in, turn them out. Pull the toes up, point the toes, spread the toes, push them into the ground. Roll the feet in, roll them out. Move your feet and ankles however you can. The second suggestion is to keep trying and don't stop. You may have to work on your feet and ankles from a sitting position. Do it. You will never regret the benefits you get for your whole body from working on your feet and ankles.

Foot massages are good too. But you have to give feedback to the giver about position, pressure and ticklishness. And if you are giving, you must take feedback and not take it personally. People with foot and ankle pain are often resistant to getting foot rubs and, just as with knees, will often anticipate discomfort before it arrives. Foot reflexology, which uses different kinds of pressure on different points on the feet, is also great for the feet, especially if you don't want a traditional foot rub. For both men and women a pedicure can be a wonderful experience. Some pedicurists are now offering reflexology as part of their services.

Waking up in the morning can be rough on us, but it can be especially tough for feet (and knees and hips as well). Before you stand on them in the morning you can warm these joints while you are still in bed. Wiggle them, flex and extend them, rotate the

29

ankles, shake them out. Actually this is also a good idea if you have been sitting for any length of time. Like anything else in our bodies they get cold and stiff when they aren't being used.

All that being said, while you are focusing and concentrating so intensely, don't forget to relax. There are surely movements that you have had fun with in your lifetime. If you find yourself motivated to dance, get silly, or otherwise reach outside of your comfort zone, and can do so safely, make the break and do it.

Starting to extend yourself physically may stir up old movement memories. When you go back to paying attention you may be surprised at what you find.

CHAPTER 4

Know and Set Your Goals

Most people who are recommended for joint replacement are experiencing pain. I would venture a guess that most people would say that their primary goal for surgery is to be pain free (or relatively so). If we think about this as an isolated goal, it could probably be accomplished with drugs. But drugs can make people dopey, may become addictive and have a whole slew of other side effects. So the goal for most people is not just to be pain free, but also to be functional.

If we follow this line of inquiry, we have to ask what does "functional" mean to the person looking for pain relief? Many people would say they want to engage in activities of daily living without restrictive pain. Some just want to be able to read or watch TV in comfort. As most pre- operative teams usually consist of the primary care provider physician, the orthopedic surgeon and the medical insurance provider; a full understanding of your personal definition of function may not be addressed.

With a little time and a bit of pressing conversation, you might remember other activities you used to do that have since been limited by your current joint pain. Should it be a goal to be able to resume that activity? Why not? And at what level? Would it be possible, post surgically, to be capable of more than you were before the development of the pain-causing condition? Why not? **Now** we're getting somewhere!

The answers to these questions are very important in goal setting and preparation for surgery. It is unfortunate that there is not a good structure in place for addressing any of these issues. This is part of what I hope to address and engage in this book.

The next section includes a questionnaire that may be helpful in learning and deciding what you want from surgery. Take time with it. If you spend a couple of weeks with these questions in mind, you will not only find your own answers, but you will come up with questions of your own. You may, or may not, have the answers. Often **just noticing** will give you a basis for conversations with your support team.

Your questions will help you decide who will be on your support team. This process should also help you learn what to ask for.

And remember...when deciding what is important to you, you can always change your mind. Just try to pay attention to why you are doing so.

GOAL SETTING AS PART OF PLANNING FOR SURGERY

➤ What is your primary purpose in having this surgery (reduce pain, increase function, prevent further injury, etc.)?

_____

_____

➤ Are you motivated more by how you feel or by how you look to others? (Has anyone made fun of you or mimicked you, called you a wimp?)

_____

_____

➤ Do you have a specific image of how you think you should look or feel? (Who are your role models, do you still see yourself as your younger self?)

_____

_____

➤ What activities give you pain now, that you want to continue doing without pain? (ex: walking, driving, dancing, bending, playing with grandchildren?)

_____

_____

➤ What activities have you stopped doing because of your current limitations that you would like to resume? (This can go pretty far back in time...)

_____

_____

➤ What have you never done that you would like to be able to do? (Have you been putting something off, like hiking, travel, ballroom or line dancing, strength training, volunteering)

_____

_____

➤ How hard have you worked with your body before? Doing what? (ex: rigorous exercise, construction work, dance classes, previous physical therapy, heavy garden/yard work)

_____

_____

➤ What is your perception of your pain tolerance? (Do you seem to feel pain like most people you know; or do you tend to feel pain intensely and others have a hard time identifying with you; or can you handle a lot of pain with little problem?

_____

_____

➢ What kind of support team do you have to encourage you? (Do you have friends, family, classmates, church members, your doctor who are patient and sympathetic?)

_____

_____

➢ What kind of support team do you have to work and play with you? (Are you close to family or friends who can comfortably be physical? Do you belong to a class or group that would like to help? Does your spouse or partner look forward to being helpful at your pace? If not, can you develop a support system now?)

_____

_____

➢ How fit do you think/feel you are overall? (Do you feel physically young or old for your actual age? Can you keep up with others at most activities you choose? Do you exercise regularly? Can you do a push up, sit up or pull up? Can you rise from a chair without using your hands?)

_____

_____

➢ What fears have you developed while living with your injury? (Going places where you'll have to walk, carrying things, icy weather, wind, walking quickly, losing your balance, etc.)

_____

_____

➢ Are you more comfortable learning and applying information yourself, or do you like to be given specific instructions?

_____

_____

➢ Do you learn better by being shown something or by hearing information; or is it best for you to actually do what you're being shown in order to learn?

_____

_____

➢ Do you see your doctor as part of your team, or as the person who knows everything that you don't know?...Or somewhere in between?

_____

_____

➢ Any other questions or answers that may have occurred to you during this process?

_____

_____

_____

_____

CHAPTER 5

What Do We Know About Pain?

All human beings, with extremely rare disordered exceptions, have and experience pain. We often assume that others understand what we mean when we talk about pain. We have as many words for describing pain as the Eskimos have for describing snow. Pain can be intense, throbbing, sharp, dull, thudding, nervy, zinging, chronic, intermittent, sudden, vague, focused, diffuse, radiating, hot, burning, numb, aching, shooting, pinching, cutting, tender, colicky, visceral, crushing... add your own.
The American Pain Foundation, in their Pain Resource Guide has developed a memory aid for describing pain - **LOCATES**

L: Location of the pain and whether it travels to other body parts.
O: Other associated symptoms such as nausea, numbness, or weakness.
C: Character of the pain, whether it's throbbing, sharp, dull, or burning.
A: Aggravating and alleviating factors. What makes the pain better or worse?
T: Timing of the pain, how long it lasts. Is it constant or intermittent?
E: Environment where the pain occurs. For example, does it occur while working or at home?
S: Severity of the pain. Use a 0-to-10 pain scale from no pain to worst ever.

See www.painfoundation.org for many excellent resources to help learn about pain and what can be done about treating it.

Most health practitioners will use the scale of perceived pain from 1 - 10 to help understand an individual's severity of pain, but this is of limited objective help because we all feel pain very differently. If you want to reduce or eliminate your pain it is useful to learn and know as much about *your* particular pain experience as you can.

Damage-indicating pain usually comes either as *acute* pain - you take a step and your hip goes, "YOW!" or *chronic* pain which is with you pretty much all of the time. An acute episode has a treatable source and is usually gone within 3 months, while chronic pain persists after an injury has healed and can go on indefinitely. Chronic pain can also come and go, but basically it is the same pain. By the time someone is having a joint replaced the pain has often become chronic, usually with acute episodes.

Having chronic pain can actually alter the way our brain and nerve pathways function. It can alter our moods, our perceptions and our responses to stimuli. Chronic pain is considered a disease in its own right. I would venture to say that responses to chronic pain are a primary obstacle to full engagement in both prehab and rehab activities.

According to the most accepted model of the role of adaptation in pain (Roy's Adaptation Model) the longer you have pain the more integrated it becomes into other aspects of your life. Some of these adaptations may be:

⚲ Getting used to the pain - Your body may become accustomed to the pain and make it feel less intense with time. The pain may also become less bearable over time.

⚲ Physical adaptations - You may change your posture by limping, for example, or by always using chair arms to help raise and lower yourself from a chair. You may modify your activities by doing less of them, exercising less, or maybe substituting one activity for another.

⋏ Emotional adaptations - These run a huge gamut and largely depend on the way you respond to stress. It is important to remember here that your emotional and physical responses to pain and stress are chemically interdependent in your body and brain. This can result in frustration, anger, moodiness, depression and resignation. Mindfulness practices like EFT, meditation and even having a healthy expressive outlet can make the difference in whether your emotional responses give you some distance from your pain or make your pain more difficult to deal with for yourself and those around you. (There are resources for these at the end of this book.)

Awareness of the adaptation phenomenon can make a difference in how we deal with the effects of pain.

What we call pain is actually what our brain "decides" the pain feels like. When any sensory stimulus reaches the brain those nerve impulses travel through several parts of the brain, including emotion and memory centers. There are numerous physical connections between parts of our brain and other parts of our bodies that determine the characteristics of the pain we feel. Pain is not "just pain," as many of us have been taught. There are many facets to pain, most of them not conscious, but we can become conscious of some of these influences.

We have *personal* and *cultural* attitudes about pain. We also have *genetic* factors that help determine not only what conditions we may be predisposed to, but also that seem to have an effect on how intensely we feel pain and what types of pain we feel most acutely, as well as how we perceive pain in the first place. There are also many *environmental* factors that influence our experience of pain. These include our *history* of pain, our *support system*, our *emotional* perceptions of our experience around the pain and our *knowledge and expectations* of our condition.

A study of Osteo Arthritis patients from Germany concluded that a variety of physical *and* psychological factors were associated with pain intensity and that appropriate pain treatment of these patients in primary care should consider as many of these factors as possible.

Culturally, we may have an understanding that it isn't appropriate to talk about pain or to complain. I grew up thinking that admitting to feeling pain for anything short of a catastrophic injury indicated that I was an inferior, weak person. Our tough American Hero images reinforce that. *Personally* some people associate pain with getting sympathy and care and they react to that association differently than others. For some, being cared for and getting attention is nurturing and accepting. For others the experience is weakening and humiliating. It is extremely difficult to keep our physical, emotional and intellectual experiences of pain separate.

We are capable of, on one hand, accepting our own pain and, on the other hand, judging another person harshly for feeling or expressing their own pain. How often have we dismissed someone who is moaning or grimacing in pain because we feel they just want attention. *We* don't express our pain that way, *we* keep it to ourselves (we think)!

That doesn't begin to take into consideration the *spiritual* ideas we can have around pain and suffering as well. Some spiritual traditions have encouraged self-inflicted pain like wearing uncomfortable clothing or engaging in self-flagellation. These are supposed to "mortify" an individual so as to keep one's mind from sinful thoughts and actions. Many people still feel that suffering is a test from God. On the other hand many meditative practices work towards removing all emotional attachments and responses to pain to lessen the overall experience of suffering. Most of us experience pain somewhere between these two ideas.

There is scientific evidence that points to *genetic* factors that affect how individuals actually perceive pain. Some evidence demonstrates that a particular gene influences not only how pain is perceived, but also has an effect on how pain is regulated. One study found evidence that variation in one gene can alter pain perception in humans. The same results were also found to be affected by a complex relationship between genetic variations in another gene, and by its relationship to other genetic factors. That same gene also appears to influence who is prone to develop common pain conditions, as well as who needs what level of opioids in the treatment of cancer pain. Another study using pressure, heat and cold, found that different individuals respond differently to different *kinds* of pain stimuli.

Interestingly, a series of studies from 2005 to 2007 indicated both that redheads have a *lower* natural pain tolerance than non-red-heads **and** that they have a *higher* pain tolerance, or that they need less anesthesia to moderate pain. So there is a lot more studying and observing to be done, demonstrating that we, as individuals, need to pay attention to and to be aware of our own patterns and needs.

Environmentally, Have you noticed, if you have joint pain, how changes in weather, altitude or location can have a very real effect on your pain level? Many studies recently have shown how the quality of our sleep affects our health. A 2009 study demonstrated that sleep-restricted subjects exhibit reduced ability to deal with their pain, whether it has to do with recognizing it, modulating it or even disengaging from it. Different types of light, including sunlight, as well as diet have also been shown to have a strong influence, not only on our general health, but also on our experience of pain.

For our purposes I think it is also important to talk about our personal *histories* of pain or discomfort. Some people with chronic, long-term pain, experience some degree of adaptation to the pain in their brains and bodies, sometimes raising their tolerance for pain, sometimes lowering it. For some the pain never feels lessened without interventions. These might include medication, meditation, or psychological or peer support.

Also contributing to our *history* of pain would be whether we have ever pushed ourselves beyond our own comfort level. Someone who's work has exposed them to extremes of heat or cold or heavy physical labor will perceive pain differently than someone who has not been challenged in this way. An athletic history where you have intentionally pushed yourself way past your comfort zone might seem like agony to a non-athlete. Unfortunately as people age and become less active, the tolerance for discomfort often fades.

My experience has shown that someone who has pushed themselves to physical discomfort voluntarily, before ever having a medical intervention, is more likely to be able to discern between pain and discomfort during rehabilitation. This is a major factor that affects successful orthopedic rehabilitation.

Engaging in a pre-habilitative movement/exercise program can stack the odds in your favor when you get to post-operative rehabilitation and physical therapy.

There is a huge *emotional* component to pain. We can begin with the understanding that it is very difficult to have pain without feeling something about that pain. Often what we feel can have a strong influence not only on how we feel our pain, but also on how we cope with it and, sometimes, on why we feel it in the first place. A lot of this is related to our histories. If we carry a lot of unresolved or unexpressed issues, our brains and hormonal systems will have learned to respond with continual stress responses that make it difficult to heal or to moderate our pain.

I'm sure you've heard the old joke; "Hey Doc, it hurts when I do this." Doc says, "Well, don't do that!" Unfortunately it is rarely as simple as that, and that attitude could even lead to failure to improve or heal the cause of the pain.

I have stated that one of the purposes of pain is to warn us of danger, but the *anticipation* of pain can have a great influence on how we actually feel pain. How often have you bumped into something and said, "ouch!" even if no pain actually occurred? Once we associate a particular movement with pain we start to modify our movements. We become afraid that the pain will recur if we do certain things. Sometimes this leads to a limp, sometimes we stop doing particular activities. Have you ever grimaced as you rose out of a chair because you expected it to hurt? A lot of times these responses and anticipations are unconscious.

Unfortunately the limitations we put on ourselves this way limit us further as often as they help us. Some of the unconscious postures can even cause tensions in parts of our bodies unrelated to the original pain. (Think about grimacing and tightening your shoulders.) Our bodies are capable of making adaptations that are helpful to us, but we also make both conscious and unconscious adaptations that can interfere with our efficient, healthy functioning.

Having a *support system* that is healthy and helpful to us in dealing with our pain and limitations can benefit our perception of the quality and intensity of our pain. This can include family and spouses, but also applies to friends, community associates and our medical treatment providers. Conversely, if the systems we rely on for support have negative feelings or behaviors, or if we perceive them as negative, they can add to our discomfort.

 Many patient advocates recommend having a second person along whenever you see a doctor. A second person should have some emotional distance from the process and can help ask and clarify questions that you have on your list, or that you haven't previously thought of. They can also help to hear and clarify responses. If there are any problems you will already have your safety net in place.

I feel that the experience of preparing for and putting together a support system can probably have a greater effect on getting to know yourself and managing your pain than any other single element in this whole process.

CHAPTER 6

Let's Understand Balance and Proprioception

Most people with orthopedic pain or arthritis have a sense of being off balance, or of having poor balance. This occurs whether your problem is in feet, ankles, knees, hips, back, shoulder, neck, even elbows, wrists and hands. So what do we know about balance? Balance can be approached within a system or between systems. This is true of the systems of the body, the physical body and its environment, and between our physical, mental and spiritual selves; as well as our social, political, emotional and intellectual selves. Take a moment to consider this. When you really think back on the times you might have had any physical mishap - whether a sprained ankle, taking a fall, or cutting yourself in the kitchen - how often might you have been rushed, irritated, or preoccupied?

I remember one time when I was much younger I was out running in New York City. I was approaching two women pushing strollers on the narrow pathway and I made several noises to let them know I was coming. They were oblivious and I got annoyed at the need to alter my pace. After I got around them I continued my mental grumbling and proceeded to twist my ankle in the worst sprain of my life!

I have seen this *off-balance* scenario play out many more times with myself as well as with others.

Here, however, we will focus on what can be done to regain physical balance and the sense that we can remain upright more often than not, especially when walking. But, as with everything else, it never hurts to examine all aspects of what makes us do what we do so that we can decide what we want to do about it.

One of the greatest correlations we see is between muscular strength and balance. You might have heard for years that poor eyesight as we age is one of the major reasons that we lose our balance or take a fall. The inner ear also has a great effect on balance, but inner ear problems usually manifest in a different way than what we are currently considering. Poor vision will have relatively little effect on our balance if we maintain the fitness of our muscles and nerves. Losing strength in our muscles, especially the leg muscles has more of an effect on balance, by far, than any other factor.

If we don't work at maintaining muscle mass and strength as we age we lose it.

Muscles have a primary effect on circulation and coordination. Using our muscles maintains strong bones. Strong, metabolically active muscles also prevent the onslaught of diabetes and the resultant loss of sensation, especially in the legs and feet. When we work our muscles consciously we maintain the neural pathways that give us faster response time. Healthy nerves also give us the feedback that allows us to know where our different body parts are in relation to each other and where we are in space without having to look or think about it. This is called *proprioception*.

Research has shown, time and again, that improving strength improves balance. It is also important to pay close attention to what you are doing and feeling (being mindful, or present) when doing strengthening exercises. The exercises included in this book are very basic. Yet virtually everyone can gain something from doing these exercises mindfully. When we pay close attention to what our bodies are doing and help them to do it we will gain strength and develop neural connections. This allows us to modify movement to get the most out of it. We will learn how to increase the difficulty when we are ready. We will learn our strengths and weaknesses and where we get in our own way.

This is another place where it is very helpful to have a support group. I strongly encourage people to put together a group, or to join an existing one for exercising, especially when doing unfamiliar movements. We can learn from others' observations and encouragement. We don't feel so alone when working with peers. We can see humor in situations and we can commiserate. Others can also help us recognize when we are making progress that we don't see.

A physical therapist or personal trainer can serve as an important piece of this support network. Keep in touch with yourself about what kind of support works best for you and remember to be honest with yourself and your network.

Proprioception

The word *proprioception* comes from Latin words that essentially mean "*sense of one's own self.*" Proprioceptive sense comes from all the signals we get from all of our other senses and lets us know where we, or parts of us, are. This sense allows you to close your eyes and still know where you are moving your arm. It allows you to walk without watching your feet. It allows us to be apparently on autopilot when doing complex tasks like driving a car (especially a stick shift) or eating while listening to conversation. Swerving at the last minute to avoid a door jamb, stepping over something with your back foot once your front foot has cleared the same obstacle, bringing your fingers together in front of you with your eyes closed - these are all examples of how proprioception works in our daily lives. *Kinesthesia* is another term for proprioception.

Our sense of balance is affected by our proprioceptive sense, and there is a generally recognizable deterioration of both as we age. The cause of this is still under study, but there are some hopeful indications. As we age we usually engage in fewer activities that build and maintain strength, flexibility, balance and endurance than when we were younger. Once activities are learned we tend to maintain an assumption that we can still do them, even years later, when we may have neglected doing those movements for a long time.

Though there is a significant quantity of research about recognizing the proprioceptive decline which occurs as most people age, there is a decided shortage of understanding or agreement on what the cause is. There seems to be a general assumption that the decline in proprioceptive sense is in great part related to the decline in physical activity, demonstrated by studies that show *active* older persons maintaining a higher sense of general proprioception than less active seniors.

As we age we often feel that we're doing things the way we always did. We recognize that we aren't as strong, as coordinated, as we once were. We experience our balance as poorer than when we were younger, but we don't often pay attention to how it is that we *do* move. Though proprioception occurs on an unconscious level developing a conscious awareness of what our body is doing and how we adapt when different needs (pain, weakness) develop can be instrumental in making us more comfortably mobile.

Even though we are usually not conscious of our proprioceptive sense (as we are usually not conscious of our senses of sight, hearing, taste, touch and smell) if we pause and think of it, we easily become aware. All of these senses can be enhanced by use and attention. Moving our bodies and paying attention to how we do so can enhance our sense of where and how we are in relation to our parts and our environment. That awareness can help us to move more effectively and to be more comfortable in our body.

CHAPTER 7

Let's Talk About Self-Image

If you read through the goal setting questionnaire, and especially if you answered many of those questions, you may have an idea of how self-image affects what we expect of ourselves. When we personally have realistic self-expectations we can better prepare for and recover from injuries and surgeries.

Realistic expectations are different for each of us and exploring them and what is behind them can have a profound impact on our overall well-being. I've observed that many of us live from our 23 year-old minds. That was probably, for most of us, when we felt pretty invincible and at the top of our physical game. We looked great, we felt great and we could do just about anything without suffering much physical discomfort. We are often surprised then, when we make a move or do an activity that "we always did without a problem" and feel stiff, sore, or worse...are completely unable to do the movement or activity.

Our culture is so youth oriented in its portrayal of the physical self that we hold on to those images of ourselves as youngsters as how we should be at our best. However, if we look at what we have done in the ensuing years, how our priorities have changed and how we chose to do things other than maintain peak fitness, we can at least honor the choices we have made. This is a part of being realistic in our view of ourselves in our current state.

We often compare ourselves to others in our age group as well. Some of us feel better in comparison and some of us feel not so good. We all have aspirations but, to be truthful, if we were serious about them we would have made a move before now. Compounded with the fact that most people don't know much about how the body works many are not currently in a comfortable position to make changes.

Or maybe we do eat healthy and exercise, but we have family that discourages us from being fit, either consciously or by having needs that limit how much time and effort we give to ourselves. Do we see this as a choice or are we victims of circumstance?

When we remember that pain is an interpretation of signals that move through several parts of our brain before we experience the conscious awareness of what we feel, we can recognize that all of our past experiences, memories and habits are in that mix. The same factors that originally formed our self-image still affect us today in everything we think, feel and do. By the same token, sometimes our conscious thoughts, feelings and memories differ from those in our unconscious.

As part of the assessment of who we are Dr. Sue Morter suggests we have a conversation with ourselves around the possibilities of what things would be like *"if I were healed and well."* What would that look like? What would you have be true in your life? Don't let your self-assessment be based on self-judgment. Take some time to breathe deep, relax, and imagine your personal energy being channeled to your best potential self. Include that in your self-image too.

To get the most out of medical interventions such as joint surgeries and replacements it is important to be as honest as possible with ourselves about *what we have, what we want and what we need.* No new joint is going to make us young again, or even make us move like we're young. But if we're honest with ourselves about who we are, how hard we are willing to work and what our support system is we can be better prepared and have more predictable results.

CHAPTER 8

Build Your Support System

The support system is the most neglected factor in preparing for, and recovering from, orthopedic procedures. The medical team will ask if you have someone at home who can attend to you and get you to physical therapy appointments after surgery or if you need to spend time in a rehab facility. Know your medical team. Make them part of your support system. Have questions for them and ask them. If what you want is not offered ask about it. Don't rush into a procedure before you feel ready.

Do ask if there is a six-week prep program (prehab) available. The likelihood there will be is very slim as I write this. You will probably get a small booklet or a few pages of a looseleaf showing a few exercises you can do using a chair or in bed. If this is all you expect to have, then ask that someone go over the exercises with you while you are doing them. There are far too many assumptions about how clear the instructions are and how the exercises work.

Ask if you can have a session with a physical therapist to go over some of the exercises in this book and to help you find which are best for you and your condition.

If you start six weeks or more before surgery on a preparatory program of exercise, movement and getting to know your physical self better, you will get some clues about your support system. Is your spouse or son or daughter going to stop what they're doing and work with you? Are they going to be encouraging and sympathetic? Or will you find them more willing to bring you food and drink in your easy chair than to push through uncomfortable movements with you? Are they constantly afraid you are going to hurt yourself instead of being mindful of your goals? Will they accept your changing yourself?

Couples tend to expect their partners to be their primary support. If the spouse is knowledgeable and experienced, this can be a good thing. If the partner is willing to learn and is open to experience, or better yet, is enthusiastic about being a knowledgeable support, this can really enhance the healing experience. However this ideal relationship is more often the exception than the rule when it comes to physical activity, exercise, prehab and rehab.

Helping someone through prehab and rehab changes relationships. If someone is willing, that's great. But get them started beforehand so everyone can be realistic about what they are capable of and willing to do. I have found it takes a *lot* of patience. Both parties need to release ego and work on communicating effectively.

Assumptions need to be dropped. This often means making an extra effort to say what you mean, as well as allowing that the other person means what they say. It is also important to ask for clarification if you're not sure what the other means, and to accept their requests for clarification without assuming they are challenging you.

Encouraging without nagging takes a special effort. Encouraging usually addresses the others' needs, while nagging attempts to address our own needs. One way to keep needs transparent is to be clear *with yourself* about what is needed, and to have options ready to get those needs met. An example of this would be to adjust the timing of an exercise session rather than being rushed.

Another example would be to admit that you're feeling impatient, vulnerable or pressured and it might be time to take a break, or to have someone else step into a particular role. Understanding the whole pain and fear-of-pain experience takes a lot of work.

This is one reason it is imperative to talk before any surgical intervention about what is expected, and what might be too much responsibility, for your spouse or partner. It is really helpful to talk about anxieties and expectations. It is important to recognize the various needs for support, and what individuals are needed, when considering a support system. When you are out of your comfort zone or field of expertise, or just tired (preferably before burn-out) it is a life-saver to be able and ready to delegate to other parts of the support system.

Even though this is a daunting challenge, I feel it is very much worth it if you are both willing to work hard at learning the physical part of what is involved and, more especially, working at communicating honestly and being flexible.

Having more than one person on your support team, however, can work exponentially better for a number of reasons. Obviously responsibility and time would be shared between several people. A change in personalities is often welcome and gives everyone a good chance to blow off steam or have a sense of humor about the others, if that helps. It can help the experience be a social time as well as work.

If you're not living with a partner, get together with your friends and talk about these issues. If they are willing and able to do so, make a schedule of who can do what support and when. This can make the difference between spending time in a rehab facility, maybe feeling abandoned on top of everything else, and feeling hopeful enough to perhaps take your recovery into your own hands and maintain continuity for your own long-term health.

Put a list on the refrigerator of anticipated needs and who can be called for help when that need arises. If friends want to help it is a gift to ask them to do so. Do this before you need to and you may find everything goes more smoothly than you thought possible.

If you can find a class with an instructor that is familiar with, and works with, people with joint pain you can find an excellent support system there. You can compare notes and encourage each other. You might even find classmates who will serve as a primary or respite caretaker for after surgery. If you don't have a class of this sort nearby, ask at your local gym or physical therapist office to see if someone is willing to lead one. Just working from this book should give anyone who is truly interested, and who has basic qualifications, enough to start with.

Engaging your support system before surgery can make post surgery rehab smoother and more successful. If you don't have enough of a support team to go home right after surgery, and must spend time in a rehab facility, have your friends or family supports visit you even when you're receiving therapy. If you're on pain medication let them know so they can adjust their expectations and perceptions of your behaviors (if it affects you that way).

It's good for others to have an idea of what you've gone through, because it is different for everyone. No one has been exactly in your shoes. And when you get to go home they can help to keep you on track with the rest of your rehab. There is no reason that these relationships can't become some of the best ones in your life.

CHAPTER 9

Tools and Resources

While most of these resources are online, the following information should be able to guide you to the right place in your local book store if books are your preference. I will try to include book titles where I have found them.

EFT or Tapping

EFT stands for Emotional Freedom Technique. It is also called "tapping." Most of the world, scientific and non-scientific, now acknowledges that we exist as whole, complex beings, rather than solely physical or emotional or spiritual. I find tapping to be an important tool for helping our inner and outer selves agree on what we want. I don't think there's anyone of rational age on the planet who has not, at one time or another, behaved in a way that got them just the opposite of what they wanted.

EFT is based on a combination of acupuncture and traditional psycho-therapeutic techniques. It entails tapping gently on several points on the hand, head and upper torso while engaging in some basic self-talk. These points are on lines that correspond to physical and energy flows in the body called meridians.

The process is easy and private and easy to learn. I recommend it because I find we often unknowingly sabotage our capabilities through our insecurities and fears. I find that tapping allows us to acknowledge what is going on with us and then to plow through and accomplish what we want anyway.

Both of these websites are excellent starting points for learning this technique.

www.eftuniverse.com   www.thetappingsolution.com

YouTube also has many videos to help you find what may work for you.

These illustrations, taken from *The Tapping Solution* and *Eft Universe*, show the basic tapping points.

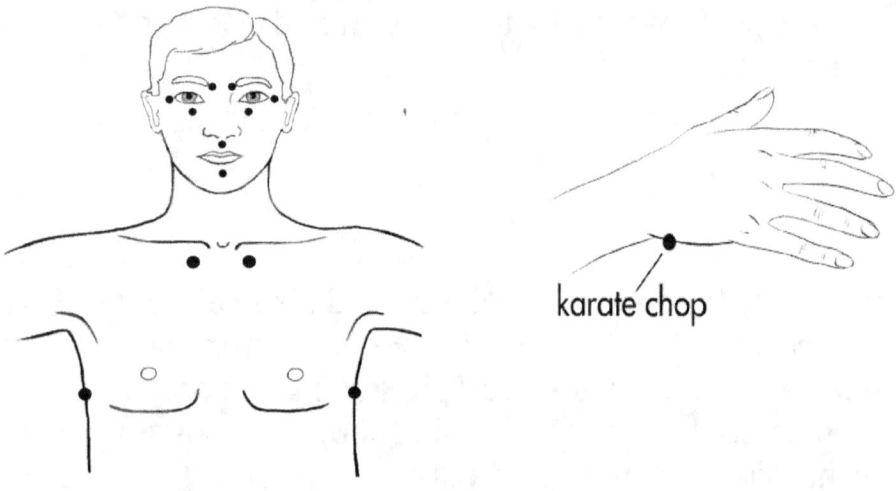

karate chop

If you're more comfortable with books you might look into:

The EFT Manual by Gary Craig

Discovering the Power of Meridian Tapping by Patricia Carrington

or even the very thorough
Emotional Freedom Technique for Dummies by Helena Fone

Massage and Other Bodywork

There are many types of massage therapies and movement therapies and as many combinations of both. The process of discerning what type might be useful can be very confusing to anyone who has not experienced them. Regardless, many of these therapies can be exceedingly helpful both pre- and post surgery. Some may help prevent, or at least delay, the need for surgery.

The Associated Bodywork and Massage Professionals website: www.massagetherapy.com has an extensive glossary of massage and bodywork techniques. It can be overwhelming. Both the ABMP and the American Massage Therapy Association: www.amtamassage.org have practitioner-finding links.

Often the best way to find a practitioner is to see who is located near you, see what style they practice, then do your research. Talking to the therapist about what they do and what their experience is, as well as sharing your concerns and needs can help you decide. Personal references can be helpful as well.

Be aware that therapies are not always what they sound like, and every therapist is different. While *sports massage* and *deep tissue* work may sound out of your league, expert practitioners at either, if it is their inclination, should be able to work with traumatized bodies without further trauma. Often Deep Tissue Massage is perceived to be "just digging in." In actuality, true deep tissue massage entails working patiently and layer by layer with great sensitivity.

Many techniques can be categorized under the more general labels of *Swedish, Acupressure and Shiatsu, Neuromuscular, Somatic and Somato- Emotional, Lymphatic* and *Myofascial.* There are also modalities like *Watsu* that take place in a warm pool.

Bodywork also includes movement therapies like *Alexander Technique, Feldenkrais Method, Rubenfeld Synergy Method, and Aston Patterning. There are many techniques that combine movement and parts of other therapies. These can all be helpful, depending on your specific needs and what is available to you.*

Physical Therapy, Personal Trainers and Group Workouts

If you have a working relationship with a physical trainer prior to surgery, you may be able to cut your physical therapy short and work with the trainer who already knows your body and who you have a trust relationship with. Though this may be more rare than not, make them a part of your team.

At some time you will work with a physical therapist. Take the questionnaire you filled out from chapter 5 to the hospital with you. Show it to the physical therapist as soon as you are introduced. It could make things go more easily and smoothly for both of you.

It might be a great idea for you to check with your local senior residential centers. They often have classes run for their residents that are led by qualified senior fitness instructors. They may or may not let non-residents participate, but more and more are expanding these programs to include the greater community.

If you are looking for a qualified *Senior Fitness Instructor or Trainer* these websites might direct you to someone local. If not, ask at your local gym or senior center if anyone is interested in becoming qualified.

www.acefitness.org - American Council on Exercise
www.ncsf.org - the National Council on Strength and Fitness
www.nasm.org - National Academy of Sports Medicine

Whether you are working on your own or with others, once you are able to take your fitness into your own hands the following websites are great resources. I've found the contributors to these sites have done a lot of work to make getting to know your body and using it well interesting and fun. They have also made the information accessible to the average person's understanding. There's something for everyone.

⊁ www.thera-bandacademy.com/exercise is the website for Theraband. They have a blog, lists and illustrations for exercises you can do at home, and a search capability that allows you to plug in what body part you are interested in and what equipment you want to use. Theraband also continues to partner with others, including researchers, who are interested in and working toward accessible fitness.

⊁ www.exercise-ball-exercises.com is an amazing website from Janice Everleigh, PT. who practices in the Toronto, ONT area. There is something here for everyone who would like to use the Swiss exercise ball for exercise. She addresses a broad spectrum of needs. Here is easy access to information, from choosing a ball, to a list of exercises by sport, and a lot of the science and reasoning between.

Ms. Everleigh recommends the books *Exercise Balls for Dummies* by LaReine Chabut and *Exercise Ball for Beginners* by Chrissie Galagher.

Exercise balls can be purchased in most department stores and in many discount stores. An air pump and instructions are usually included in the package. A general guide for size is:

Under 5' tall	45cm	5'0" to 5'6"	55cm
5'7" to 6'0"	65 cm	over 6'0"	75cm

Whether your legs are shorter or longer relative to your body is more important than your height. Many places only have 55 and 65 cm balls, as either will serve well for most people.

The more you weigh, the firmer the ball should be filled to support your weight.

- www.lifelongexercise.com - is a good website to get a start on taking control of your personal fitness.

- http://www.somatics.com/walking.htm - a good resource for general information about walking effectively. The home page treats the topics of pain, movement patterns, stiffness, balance, errors of improper movement and thinking, chronic tension patterns and exercises.

- http://www.sitandbefit.org/home - I discovered the Sit and Be Fit program on PBS television. It may seem basic, but is based on good science and a good understanding of the needs of people who are at a very basic level of fitness. The workouts are available on DVDs.

- http://www.swingwalker.net - If you want to see how the body walks best in a natural, pain free manner, check out the short videos on this website from a series of researchers. It really helped me see what was in my head.

- www.painfoundation.org - The website for the American Pain Foundation offers a wealth of information that is helpful to health workers and laypersons alike. The APF is a nonprofit with the mission to educate, support and advocate for people affected by pain.

GLOSSARY

Acute Pain - Immediate pain with a treatable source that usually lasts less than three months.

Chronic Pain - Pain that persists after an injury has healed, and which can be constant or intermittent, and can go on indefinitely.

Core - As relates to the body, "the core" refers to central muscles in the area of lower stomach, low back, hips and pelvic floor, as well as the "belt" of abdominal muscles that keep us upright.

Dystonia, kinesthetic - A general ignorance about body movement and everything related to it.

EFT - Emotional Freedom Technique, also known as Tapping: A technique based on a combination of acupuncture and traditional psycho-therapeutic techniques. The technique can be done with a practitioner or alone and entails tapping on several points on the body while engaging in some basic self-talk.

Femur - The long bone of the thigh.

Gluteus Muscles - The muscles we generally consider the buttocks: the gluteus maximus, gluteus minimus and the gluteus medius. These are the largest and strongest of the muscles that help balance our hip and leg movements. The g. Maximus, along with the hamstrings, pulls the leg backwards from the hip (extension).

Hamstrings - The three muscles in the back of the thigh that help extend the hip and bend the knee. They are named the semitendinosus, semimembranosus and the biceps femoris.

Ilium - The pelvic bone we generally think of as our hip bone.

Iliofemoral Joint - What we think of as the "hip joint," where the thigh bone (Femur) connects into the ilium of the pelvis.

Ischium - The lower part of the pelvis that includes the pubis and the sitz bones.

Kinesthetics - The study relating to our perception and awareness of our bodies in motion, and of our body movements. Often interchanged with proprioception.

KQ - Kinesthetic Quotient - Physical intelligence about one's own body.

Pelvic Floor Muscles - Also referred to as the pelvic diaphragm, and part of what we call our *core* muscles; the levator ani, pubococcygeus, iliococcygeus and coccygeus muscles.

Plasticity - The ability to be molded or changed.

Prehab - Short for prehabilitation - A recently coined term used to identify the process of treatment and education that prepares *in advance* for surgical or other medical procedures. According to the Theraband website Hygenicblog.com (one of the first to use this term) prehab "refers to the exercise performed before surgery that helps reduce functional decline after surgery."

Rehab - Short for rehabilitation - the process of treatment and education that lead to recovery from disease, injury or medical procedure.

Preloading - Stimulating a muscle to contract in order to resist or control a weight (including bodyweight) before the actual exercise begins.

Proprioception - The awareness of our body posture, movement, and position based on input from our sensory and neurological systems.

Quadratus Lumborum - A muscle of the lower back which goes from the top of the hip bone (ilium) to the bottom rib and the first four lumbar vertebrae. The quadratus lumborum helps bend the body to one side when standing, and is very important in helping lift and move each hip as we walk.

Quadriceps - The four muscles on the front of the thigh that help flex the hip and straighten the knee. They are named the rectus femoris, vastus lateralis, vastus intermedius and the vastus medialis.

Sitz Bone - The nickname for the ischial tuberosity, which is the bony bump on the pelvis we feel through our buttocks when we sit.

Sacrovertebral Joint - The joint at the bottom of the lumbar spine where the spine connects to the sacral bone of the pelvis.

Sacrum - The pelvic bone at the back that ends in the tail bone (coccyx).

Somatic - Relating to the physical body.

Sports Medicine - The branch of medicine relating to sports training and and athletic performance and injuries. It differs from other medicine in that it aims for maximal, instead of adequate, performance and efficiency.

Squat - A traditional exercise where one starts from standing and, remaining as upright as possible, bends the legs to move into a sitting or squatting position. This can be done through a small or great range of motion, according to the abilities of the individual.

Tai Chi - A traditional Chinese exercise system, consisting of a series of self-paced movements which flow smoothly into one another. Tai Chi can be performed alone or in a group, standing or seated.

Tapping - See EFT.

Visualization - Mentally imagining or rehearsing an activity, including every aspect of the activity or movement that one is able to use in the imagining.

INDEX

American Pain Foundation 37, 60
Anatomy Trains i
Balance and strength 45
Balance and vision 45-46
Common physical issues
      abdominals... 27-28
      ankles and feet............... 29-30
      arthritic hands............... 24
      clothing... 23
      immobile hips.............. 26-27
      knees 28-29
      low back.. 24-26
      pain in the standing leg.............. 27
      stiff neck 23
      weak shoulders 24
EFT...25, 55-56
Exercises
      back leg raises 9
      balance ball sit 15
      floor hip walk 17
      hip hike 10
      hip wheels 11
      huddle stretch 13
      knee raises 7
      neck rotations and sidebending............... 5
      pelvic tilts, standing 4
      rise from chair 16
      seated legs lift............................... 12
      shoulder set 11
      spider... 12
      toe raises/calf stretch...........................3
      torso rotations 6
      wall plank..................................... 14
      walk in place 13

Joints and muscles work together 20, 23
Kinesthesia 47
Kinesthetic dystonia ....i-ii
KQ-kinesthetic quotient..................................... i
LOCATES 37
Massage 56-57
Morter, Dr. Sue 50
Myers, Thomas... i
Pain
      acute... 38
      adaptation to 38-9
      adaptations and attitudes
            anticipation.. 43
            cultural 39-40
            emotional 42
            environmental 41-42
            genetic 41
            spiritual 40
            support system 43
      chronic 38
      describing 37
Physical therapist 22,47,51,53,58
Proprioception 46
Roy's Adaptation Model 38
Thompson, Eli ii
Visualization 22